SOCIAL MISFIT

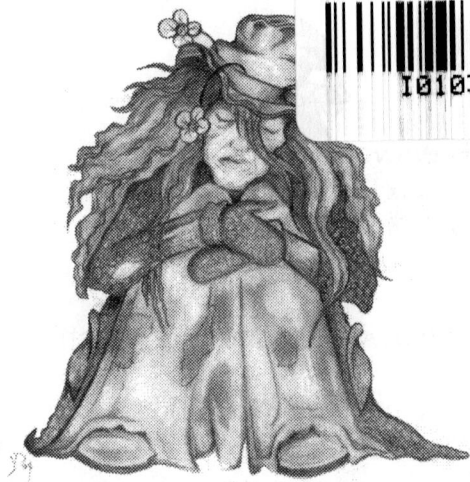

A COLLECTION OF POEMS
BY
DEBRA C RUFINI

Published by:
Chipmukapublishing
PO Box 6872
Brentwood
Essex
CM13 1ZT
United Kingdom

http://www.chipmunkapublishing.com

First published in 2000.
This edition 2006.

Copyright © 2006 Debra C Rufini

ISBN: 978 1 84747 020 1

About the Author

Urged to deal with hard hitting issues in written form, Debra C. Rufini is sensitive towards such matters of mental health, suffering, pain, depression, confusion, intolerance, people's emotions and experiences.

As a qualified Hypnotherapist/Psychoanalyst and ex-Samaritan, she truly appreciates the need for encouragement as opposed to rejection.

She believes that each personality is formed through the ingredients of opinion, decision, life's experiences and circumstances, some being more unfortunate than others.

This volume should be read with concern and empathy for the victims it involves.

Foreword

'Each true personality is formed through the ingredients of opinion, decision, life's experiences and circumstances. Some characters are happy, some are sad, some are sane and some are mad. Others are concealed, whilst others are revealed'

Outcast, Reject, Misfit, Different, Weird, Eccentric. Those who don't conform to the 'norm'.

People create 'Social Misfits' through Society's prejudiced nature, which can lead to low self esteem, an incorrect judgement on how one really views oneself, a limit on what one's capabilities are, not to mention desperation, suicide and so on. The 'sticks and stones' deception could not be more untrue!

This book contains poems dealing with the issues faced by (created) Social Misfits and those who bear a burden which is built by mental bruising. Its aim is to open eyes to the awareness of victimisation.

SOCIAL MISFIT

Contents

1 The Big Bruise Show

Meeting for the embryo.
Forming fast, progressing slow.
Gaining what is rightfully yours.
No decision past first course.
Choice for life was never made.
Its price by you has to be paid.
Whether you like it or you don't,
you've no part in your existence vote.
Forced out of the safe cocoon.
No more time left in the womb.
Time to face the universe.
Could there be anything worse?

When she shot me out, she died.
No Mummy to be Mother's pride.
Born without my sight or limbs.
Born a Down's Syndrome victim.
Born with a positive HIV test,
through the old woman's foolishness.
Have to face life with my stomach churned.
Why did she have to meet the sperm?

Here I am, and infantile,
mischievous and pretty vile.
Wanting to get my revenge
upon existence that offends.
Have to meet some more of me.
Have to make out I'm happy.
Have to mix and socialize.
Have to wear this constant disguise.

Watching happy faces play.
Wanting just to get away.
Wanting to not be part of them.
Wanting to return to the womb again.

Having to start school today.
Here we go again this way.
This time will be ten times worse.
This time it's not been rehearsed.
Living life played by the rules.
Lessons in becoming fools,
dodges themes to influence
children of indifference.
Later, to extend this bad dream,
life is smashed to smithereens.
Welcome in, you puberty.
Have you got something nice in store for me?

So goodbye then, you childhood.
Hello, monthly gush of blood.
What purpose have you for me then?
I'm a confirmed lesbian.
I'll take the shit from society,
but don't expect my apology.
My college's gay union
allows only men called Julian.
Studying to qualify.
Studying to just scrape by,
in this screwed up house of thugs,
whose chewed up brains are filled with drugs.

Leaving college with no goal,
but to only end up on the dole.

Got myself a relationship
with a two-timing woman not prepared to
commit.
Family disapprove some more.
Drinking to make sense of it all.
Working merely to get sacked.
Homeless, skint and getting fat.

Marrying to hide preference.
Battering, he loves to punch.
Admitted to the whacked wives home,
where we provide the 'big bruise show'.
That's where I began recovery,
until he interfered with me.
Soon after, hit the tragedy
of the shooting of my direct family.
Once for release, but now to replace.
This time, with the den of the mental case.

Banging heads on padded divisions.
Screaming for no-one else to listen.
Entered young to exit old.
Shoved around, do what I'm told.
They now inform me of a niece,
but I'm sure all my kin have deceased.
She's pleased I'm here at my expense,
longing for her inheritance.

So I've popped my pills – won't be long now.
My remains up for grabs by the greedy cow.
A life, death and suicide victim.
Born with a head start lose, destined not to
win.

So I've just popped under ground for a
permanent break that's called to die.
Thank God I can't pop 'round again, to wave
my last goodbye.
Life is one deep wound where you can never
bathe the sore,
and the answer's always no, when asked; is
it really worth it all?

2 Thelma Fews

A Church's fond memory of tragedy seems
rare.
"He will not beyond us that limit to bear".
A Mother, a Daughter, an Actress's smile,
sat in the back pew for only a while.
A Mother, a Daughter, a Wife,
shared in a role of all three.
A time to be selfish,
to be spared for the desperation key.

A child so observant could sense the tense
strain,
although the undeveloped cannot place their
finger on pain.
Grown ups were supposed to be happy and
full of the cross.
Not vacant and starey, like she always was.
Grown ups were supposed to be happy and
blessed, even in their loss.
Her lacking in something, her life did it cost.

Now, I thought that you had to always put on
the lid,
and pull down the blinds, when this foreigner
hit.
And I thought the done thing was for grown
ups to hide,
Should a face ever appear absent in having
Jesus at it's side.

What does it take to reach for that state of
mind,
of kissing the grave, and wishing for closing
time?
Differing tragedies all amount to the same.
Their level in sickness doesn't alter the pain.
Candyfloss life is for only the dense.
Razors are given to those experienced.

Thelma, it's not until now that I understand.
The years have passed by, and I see now
life's plan.
Thelma, I know that your Master within,
has taken you back for REAL life to begin.

So, in her life now, I believe that she's free,
from troubles and muddles and overall
catastrophe.
How I wish that I could have saved your
suicide.
My age and your mind were not enough to be
applied.
So Thelma, I look forward to meeting with
you.
I'm sorry I misunderstood back in the pew.

3 Another News Headline

Just another day when the papers arrive.
Another journey on my heavy pushbike.
Another long school day put behind me.
Another road for my delivery.

Another farmyard of the familiar kind.
Another letterbox with no-one behind.
Another end of day that takes you by
surprise.
Another batch of men up to no good in
disguise.

Another victim held to the wrong place and
time.
Another shooting fired to end this life of mine.
Another news headline, one of many we've
read before,
on another paper's page, which I can no
more shove through your door.

Another thirteen year old of innocence.
Another group of criminals imprisoned for
their offence.
Another young boy deprived of a lifetime's life
ahead.
Another curse I throw up from this grave
which leaves me dead.

Just another crime the law accused on the
four mistakes.

Another roof protest to stress the extreme of
this piss take.
Eighteen years is a long time to be
imprisoned for burglary.
Convicted for the killing,
now seems a murder's mystery.

4 Poor Guy!

Here he is,
dressed up to the nines.
Not the type of toy
your kids would cuddle in bed.
It's queer this.
A tradition granted as fine.
Celebrating the fact
one's human life is now dead.

Here he sits,
slumped against a wall,
wearing a babygro,
he's got a football for his head.
It's the pits.
His crime was one so small,
when compared to those which
actually took place instead.

If he were
here today,
the poor guy would be
left with an inferiority complex.
Once a year,
we bring him out for money,
so that we can kill him
at a barbecue's innocence.

5 Hunger

If you go out in the woods today,
you're in for a big surprise.
If you go out in the woods today,
your Grandma will have big eyes.
There's Goldie on her every day way,
but on this journey, she's having to pay,
for today's the day the wolfman will have his
picnic.

There was hunger all through the forest,
yet it was so peaceful if you were deceived
into being honest.
You would think just by one glance that it was
such an awesome scene,
but terror made the wood unclean.

The piggies peered out through their window
from their little hut.
They knew by now that they had to always
keep the doorway shut.
They spotted petite Goldilocks happily
skipping along,
singing on her merry way, her merry little
song.

The piggies all three asked where she was
skipping to head for.
She showed them cakes for Grandma who
felt very sick and poor.

"I must be on my way now, for Grandma will
worry if I'm late".
The piggies screamed out loud for her to stop
and hesitate.

"Don't take that short cut Goldie, through that
dangerous part of land.
Grandma, if you're a little late, will surely
understand.
It's best to get you safely there, than not get
you there at all.
You can't arrive with blood-stained clothes at
Grandma's chained up door".

Goldie snapped back at the piggies, all the
closet bound three.
"I'll take that short cut if I want to, it's my
territory.
Rules can't be set to not walk through the
woods, just because it's dark.
It's a free wood, just as the free trees have
their free share of bark".

So the piggies with their pal, Goldie, all
female four,
decided to not be overruled and live secluded
any more.
"Who's afraid of the big bad wolf", was sung
hand in hand,
for all the sisters of the neighbourhood wood
to continue and understand.

Goldie left the piggies, knowing that her seed
was wisely sown.
She reached for Grandma's house, where
she was surely not alone.
A lot of commotion she heard, before
answered was the door.
A hairy beast dressed in drag left
Grandma's feet dangling out of the drawer.

"Grandma, what staring eyes you have, and
teeth so sharp and big.
You've changed your hairstyle once again, or
is that yet another wig?
Hey Grandma, you don't usually hold my
hand with such a grip so strong.
Oh Grandma, I really guess that I should
have seen straight through you all along".

Goldie made it out the back so fast, and
scarpered through the trees.
Wolfman caught her right up, when she
tripped and fell to her knees.
He jumped out, such a hard man, in such a
bad attitude,
ordering the blond chick to fulfil him in his evil
mood.

He said:
"There's one thing that I must rob from you to
make me so very pleased".
She said:
"Don't beat around the bush,

and don't let that be my precious gift of
virginity".
Now, everyone knows that female existence
is only here to defeat,
and everyone knows that big bad wolves all
need their luscious meat.

"So open up your flap, and let me invite
myself in,
or I'll huff and I'll puff, in spite of my lack of
warm welcoming.
Doesn't this make you feel good, my little
golden haired princess?
Just be thankful I'm not your Brother, or this
would be classed as crime of incest".

Goldie was left to stagger to her feet from her
back.
There was no sign of the beast now, of the
vicious attack.
"Grandma, Grandma, I can't afford it to not
be you this time".
"Hold on Dear, while I squeeze out of this
bottom drawer of mine".

"I don't quite know what happened now, but I
dreamt about a big dog or big bear.
I must have sleep walked and ended up here,
when you first appeared there.
I'm so sorry to have missed you.
Hey, what's that eruption in my lunch?"
"Oh Grandma, that is nothing compared to
the volcano in my cunt!"

"I must run on back, to tell the piggies my
event of the day".
"You really asked for it after all", is what they
all three will say.
I'm really sure that we request big bad
wolves, when we freely take a stroll,
and that every big bad wolf is each girl's
dream, to fulfil her essential role.

There is hunger all through the
neighbourhood,
and it's a very peaceful place if you have
misunderstood.
You would think just by one glance, that the
streets viewed such a comfortable scene,
but terror makes their name unclean.

6 I Am Hungry For My Faith That's Turned

They've brought me here.
These few I call friends.
How I trust them.
My age in years they've lived again,
so they have taken me under their wing.
I'm confused and naive to this new scene.

My whole life long,
it's true I've preferred the crowd
of advanced years.
My teenage era's not proud
of a simple misfit, as I stand.
But this adult's party,
is it not out of hand?

I am hungry
for my faith that's turned,
so I'm wondering,
should I play concerned?
All these drugs before my eyes.
Is their intake really wise?

I feel dizzy
amidst distorted sound.
Twisted laughter
I can hear all around.
Any more, my mind's blanked out,
apart from wanting just to shout.

Four hours later,

I awake from sleep.
A dazed recalling
of that strange tasting drink.
I am sore in my arm and my arse.
I wish to know,
but they're not fit to ask.

So I'm sat here
in the waiting room chair,
requesting too much,
but the answer's not there.
The result's reply makes me scream:
Semen up my rectum and heroin in my
bloodstream.

Am I an object
to be taken advantage of?
My feelings are vulnerable.
Where are these friends who support and
love?
Where does this leave my trust
with the responsible age matured?
Infected life is my only fact assured.

7   Needles In The Sand

We all did heroin in the sea,
then threw our needles into the sand.
You should always remember those
who remember you – and?!

The drizzly blue sky
held us all in its arms.
It swore to safely
protect us from any harm.

Bound in togetherness,
our caring family
secured every forearm
as firm as tight could be.

I'm not really me,
I'm an extension of you.
I'm burning in your head.
I'm the pounding kangaroo.

We all took heroin in the sea,
then threw our needles into the sand.
You should always consider those
who consider you – and ?!

8 It's Only A Joke

Well, his character is wild, and his humour is felt,
but sometimes he can probe too far below the belt.
He jokes about sex abuse and stillborn babies,
racism and filth, and scared raped ladies.

Well, does he know that these worldly happenings really do go on?
While he is sharing his wit, the Pakistani is rubbing himself clean,
hoping that one day soon, his dirty colour will be gone.
The stillborn baby has died, failing to make his unknown dream,
and as for the scared raped lady, just as much fun filled the scene.

Well, all that he can do here is seem to laugh.
He claims that it's only a joke within his sense of humour wacky and daft.
Does he understand that such an event really doesn't lack?
While he is telling his incredibly funny gag,
his subjects for amusement are victims under attack.

9 Carrie

Well, you suffer all their mockery and
torment,
as they cruelly tease the way that you've
turned out.
Second class are you to their flock who are
all sent
to be burnt out.

As you approach womanhood there in the
shower,
your naive mind believes that you will bleed
to death.
You're displayed by their control for the evil
power
which you'll invest.

Your Religious Mother never wants to let you
go,
yet your Star Tutor wants you to be set free.
You're the victim, be their purpose to help or
hinder,
or to believe.

As he shocks you with his invite to the prom
night,
as his partner, it's all too good to be true.
Where's the catch for the best evening spent
in your life?
Where's the clue?

When they vote for you as Queen of the
whole dance floor,
and you're stood up on that stage with pride
to glow,
that tin bucket filled with pig's blood pelts
down on you,
drenched from head to toe.

What a sick joke to be played at such an
event,
where perfection only yearns for just a while.
Sweet revenge will have them pay
and have them prevent those wicked smiles.

If they're jumping into flames, they're sure to
get burnt.
So my guess is that it's what you have to do.
Wipe them out, as they did not grasp what
they should have learnt
from the example of you.

So they've hit the road heading to stoke the
fire,
leaving one behind, screaming nightmares
every night.
Both parties fulfilled each relishing desire,
claiming their right.

Now, your Mother, she regrets your birth's
arrival.
So she tries to take your life, to take you
back,

but your Supernatural mind won't have her
knife you,
so you attack.

Carrie, stay there midst the rubble and the
debris,
Carrie, lay there underground and
undisturbed.
Carrie, say to me that you're more than a
memory
who left unheard.

10 Jan

So I've arrived here with my nerves inside
out,
waiting for a glimpse of what this fixation's all
about.
You came and took me by surprise.
You made fantasy come true.
From the window I looked right in your eyes.
I was so near to being near you.

I know you're not up for grabs, but I none the
less adore you.
I was smitten with awe from the first time that
I saw you.
Keep thinking how I'd like to spend this week,
yet wishing I'd never come here.
They say your heroes you should never
meet!
So out of reach, but yet so near.

When my dreams get wild, well they get so
out of hand.
But then they're only for I alone to
understand.
Now we don't know each other, you and I.
I wish I could call you my friend.
All good things must end, as I wave goodbye.
I wish that I could see you again.

These sweet memories that never even knew
you,

yet had ideas, who knows? They could have
been true.
This image of a woman I'd never see again,
but would never forget.
Yet as fantasy after all, it had to remain,
if only to protect.

So you won't be out there for me to bump
into now.
Maybe one day I'll willingly warn you of this
good pal.
Well it's been a while since I was there.
How I wish I could have talked to you.
I've pulled away so far to be fair.
How I wish I could have walked up to you,
if only to say 'goodbye' and 'thank you'
for making my dream come true!

11 Alien Abuse

I'm as sane as the next man.
I've never strayed from my mind.
I have a cosy home,
and family so fine.
I had a bad nightmare,
a one off dream to forget.
They gave me a comfy chair.
They gave me anal sex.

I met a real life scream.
I met a strange, strange man.
He took me to his place,
where I met with his clan.
They messed with my backside,
to sort our differences out.
I pleaded with him, this time
to call my kids for help.

It shook me night after night.
I, stolen from my family.
I missed my bedside wife,
each nightly tragedy.
I did not request their peculiar company.
What does this reveal about my name?
One by one they appeared in their flock to
greet me.
Is this me who is going insane?

I'm on my journey again.
They insert a wire into my head.
Can you feel pain in a dream,

or merely within life instead?
I saw an expert man
who confirmed it's reality in truth.
He confessed that I've in fact become
another victim of alien abuse.

12 Unconscious Living

It occurred to me again last evening.
Woken up when my teeth were soft.
Recognizing those playful armchairs.
Those clean stains had been all washed off.

I awoke, weighing five foot seven.
Those green lines ditched me once again.
I ran past those deer, way behind me.
In the flood, I was drier than the rain.

Snoring candyfloss into the brain.
The world can spin, I've forgotten my map.
I met a little goose on the way to the huge
marshmallow.
Distorted reflections of my paperback.

Where does it say one should dwell only on
the outward?
I'm so in love with my inward dream.
The uncontrolled state of unconscious living
cannot be denied, when from it released.

I once dreamt of my life's one passion,
I once slept to reach reality.
If cast aside was my illusion life,
what hope would I have of a life pleasing to
me?

Freedom enters when our minds are resting.

All that can't be lived out of life can be lived
here.
Twisted around with crazy differences,
but when else would we burst free from our
giant tear?

13 The Shepherd Of The Funny Farm

My mind's in confusion,
as still as revolving doors.
My firm decision can't decide,
for it's so honestly false.
I live one day at a year.
I lose my way when I steer,
whenever I go driving in my little pogo-
sticking horse.

Eyes looking at me
wherever I stare,
when I go to steal my weekly shopping
at the silent fun fair.
Then I return home to hum and rock to my
only known tune,
in the privacy of my cosy and small white
padded room,
where I can punch my head and pull out my
hair.

I never feel sad.
I'm always depressed.
My every day life is lived
in its every way best.
My friends and I are so happy
living up here in our close knit distant cuckoo
tree.
I wouldn't say that my life is in any state of
mess.

Observing my surroundings,

there goes another passing me by.
How can I ever get to talk to
all these racing pigs in the sky?
The man below me looks down.
His head is raised up to the ground.
I'd never want to live under his permanent
sigh.

Here come those questions again,
those ones that I can't hack.
I'm feeling just about ready
for yet another attack.
Don't pluck me out from my pie.
My pastry ceiling kindly wants to protect me
from a world where I'd only have to try,
and a world where after reaching so far
forward,
would only be pulled back.

So now if you'll excuse me,
I must be on my way.
I have to steal this awesome situation,
for I'm not willing to pay.
Now a sigh of relief you can breathe,
while you thank God you're not me.
But if you were,
what would your critics have to laugh about
or say?

Is this a problem for you?
Please then let me explain:
The more you curse it's sensitive nature
down,

the more I give you it's blame.
Your cruel and unfair affect on me
has turned me senseless and loopy,
with your own opinion which selfishly states
that I am the one insane.

Don't go and avoid me.
Don't be alarmed.
I'm never dangerous or threatening.
I don't mean you any harm.
You've got your view of distorted me all
wrong,
and although I don't belong,
I'm still the shepherd of my flock
back home in my funny old farm.

Judging from the outside
without looking at the in,
however can you know exactly what's going
down
at a place where you've never been?
Don't look now,
but you're looking kind of stupid,
standing by society's stated standards for
normality
which in us are so deeply rooted.
So stand aside, while we belt out to cry
from what cracks us up behind our emotional
screen.

So please then do excuse us
when we feel the need to break free.

We somehow don't ever appear to be
ashamed
of showing response in any form to whatever
we see.
Our expressions to you may seem far more
than strange,
but we are only climbing free from our cage.
And maybe it would do you good
to be emptied out to make room for insanity.

When you're bursting at the seams,
you have to let off steam.
If you try your hardest to control it,
you'll only erupt as you try to console it.
Better let out than kept in.
A waterfall shouldn't ever have to fake
and keep under control it's full powered
energy,
for the sake of society's expected calm
and steadily flowing stream.

14 Eccentric Old Bid (Loopy Lottie)

Many claim that she's lost it,
with her ideas that don't fit
their so-called 'normality'.
A lonely outcast's the outcome –
named 'Loopy Lottie', the odd one.
They're scared to peep outside of sanity.

Her presentation may seem strange.
Her manic grey hair forms a long mane.
Her red shoes are too big for her feet.
Green socks and on her hat, flowers.
They stand laughing at her for hours.
Their amusement act is incomplete.

Since a child, she's been rejected.
Now, old age only wants to be accepted.
She's not asking for as much as to be liked.
Even adulthood faces mockery;
"Something I thought by now would have left
me,
but no, it's clinging on with all it's might".

She shouts it out in the High Street;
"I'm mad, and you're sat in my seat",
as they cross over to the other side.
As the centre of their attention,
she doesn't care much for prevention.
She's happy for them to stare with mouths
and eyes wide.

They play their least part to support her.

This neighbourhood disturbed would much
rather abort her.
Can't they see their entertainment needs to
give help a try?
"This world will shrink thin and I'll grow wide,
then I will leave by jumping off its side",
she yells, as they fail to grasp how the
problem with them lies!

15 Queen Socialiser

She was crowned as Queen Socialiser.
Her popularity gained her many a friend.
She'd walk out from the crowded disco,
to hide in a corner where she would never be
spotted again.
She would need her 'alone' moment,
where she could be allowed to escape from
all surrounding,
where she never had to fulfil expectations,
but only find space to lock herself in.

As the days passed by,
they noticed how less and less time she
seemed to spend with them.
Now, whenever they will call her,
she seems to act strange and 'round the
bend.
She's become very cold and distant.
Some would say that she's gone loopy.
So now she's been admitted to a hospital
where the white coated men are all so
friendly.

Her folk now are understanding,
and it's only now that they realise
that this took it's gradual process,
which came to her, as much to them as such
a big surprise.
Yet only three short months ago
she would have laughed about the person
she's now become,

only due to the fact that her sanity
had to break to come undone.

Her folk will see her through this.
They will be her strong supportive backbone.
They will comfort and confirm her with the aid
of their love,
that she doesn't have to face this confusing
situation alone.
They are determined to bring her out
of her present disturbed state of mind.
This is what she needs foremost now:
true friends who are patient, willing and kind.

At a crisis point in one's life,
who would they depend on to turn to?
It would never happen to them,
just as it could never happen to you.
A friend or close companion
wouldn't fail their loyalty and love
by abandoning the matter,
giving up and walking away.
The longer left without the essential help,
the longer their situation will stay.

16 Face Value (Display Me Distorted)

Your mind's eye looks through maturity,
to not see difference,
but see acceptance.
You shine the face value of purity,
through a child of innocent pre-adolescence.

When your judgemental age has crept up on
you,
your view of me now
will be aborted.
Though your same eyes will you see me
through,
somehow their mind will display me distorted.

My outward appearance will determine
how worthy a person I am in your eyes,
when you grow up to be
a small-minded bundle
of bored insecurity.
And it won't be until if or when
you decide to mature again,
that you'll get to see otherwise,
when you learn how to live,
and when you get a better view of me.

Granted will be
your wish to rebel, pathetically.
You'll follow with the sheep,
only to get sheared.
You've the cheek to curse at me
your applicable terminology.

Juvenile personality
has no room to interfere.

The babe wins first prize for maturity.
The most sincere,
the least intellectually clever.
In second place the adult stands
where the winner theoretically should be,
and the loser adolescent's growth
is nearly always never.

17 Ten Minutes 'Til Closing Time (The Wailing Jim)

Ten minutes 'til closing time
comes around again.
He gets up.
Standing on the bar,
he wails his tone deaf sound again.
They get het up.
His audience more abusive than not,
insists to him to stop.

As far as his crowd's concerned,
all that they can see,
as the outsiders looking in,
is a drunkard,
attention seeking who will never be
in life to win.
Taking him at face value alone;
He 'struts his stuff' upon his throne!

Never to terminate,
the cancer brings the tear.
His motive of song
is wanting to make up
for those he's grieved, by cheer
before he's gone.
They moan about and put him down.
They have no idea about this clown.

Ten minutes 'til closing time
comes around again.

Three months on,
the crowd is half expecting
Jim to wail his tone deaf sound again,
despite he's gone.
You never know what you miss until it goes,
and boy, at this bar does it show!
So re-named is the pub in memory of him:-
'The Wailing Jim'.

18 A Place For The Fish Bone

She lived only for her own self.
A rich old lady with no time.
Love was lacked,
as much as gain was plenty.
Always ignored was the door bell's chime.
Never a third foot ever
stepped past the welcome mat, as it stood so
dead.
Never a place laid at the table
for an extra meal time head.

Her home, the local kids played its castle,
though their fantasies didn't live.
Their minds were inside,
whilst hers was genuinely dining.
Choked on a fish bone:
Three weeks to live.
"What's the point of all of this?"
was the question on her mind.
Death will tear me from my huge life's hut.
Death will leave all this behind.

So was brought to life what never
any soul ever dreamed to exist.
Good deeds and company entertained in
their hundreds.
Now wondered why all once was missed.
"The very least that I can do now,
is to enjoy myself with these young pups".
Joined them on her large bed, bouncing,
when she coughed her fish bone up.

Due to her such change in spirit,
she saved life, whilst giving it too.
Maybe damaged were her possessions,
but which would you have chosen to do?
Changed from keeping into sharing.
Life gained through her own merit.
Now her lesson was learnt preparing
all she did and will inherit.

19 Dear Jeevis

It was ever such a lovely day,
in that little village very far away.
The family Jeevis with their servant, Grace,
on their tour around to check out the sights of
this place.

Was very cosy, yet not very used to.
They were almost human for once.
There was no such show, for it was only
those few,
away from society of the upper kind.
For just one moment in time they left all
falseness behind.

A family nearby, as they always do,
came up to greet the ones who appeared to
be new.
Should the Jeevis family now act above, to
show just who they are?
They were now faced with paupers, who
were the lowest here by far.

The snobbery at first got in the way,
but it wasn't long before they could cope with
their kind of day.
They soon became the closest of the
friendship kind.
After all, they were only the visitors having to
leave all offishness behind.

The children play, while the adults talk and
natter.
Yes, they were human too, despite their lack
of grammar.
They went out, they stayed in, their house
became their home.
They accepted every condition and not once
did they moan.

Taking to their lifestyle of dirt and sweat.
Well after all a holiday must have to be
adaptably met.
The Jeevis's not too familiar with the
surroundings here,
consequently found father Jeevis sinking into
a bog too near.

The Jeevis's like almost any other time,
had to go on ahead, leaving the paupers way
behind.
They all pulled away not attempting to get
Mr Jeevis out. They all just cried through
upset.

The waiting for the pauper family,
was only a matter of ten seconds preciously
to see.
They came running, and they knew exactly
what to do,
as they went on ahead and rescued him,
unlike the spectating few.

Well, the fun seemed so endless that was
enjoyed by them all,
but the time came all too soon for their
returning call.
They agreed to writing about their friendly
terms,
but there was a lesson here that the Jeevis's
should have learnt.

Back to the scene of snobbery and inhuman
acts.
The family to their true lifestyle were now
brought back.
The adults talk in the upper fashion,
while the children play with no sticks or
stones,
but with some toys with action.

All was soon forgotten of their holiday.
They never told any of their friends.
Well, they were only paupers anyway.
To the other side, it was their highlight of life,
to have such visitors come to see them there
in their light.

The Jeevis' ball was to take its place,
on an evening so cool with nothing to
disgrace.
What incident could ruin such a happy time?
Not a knock at the door, with some peasants
behind.

A face should have seen such a welcome sight,
but instead of which, met with a "go back" bite.
After pleading with the butler to let them come in.
After succeeding in telling their friendship with the Jeevis's was convincing.

"Mr. Jeevis", a cry came to halt
all that was going on, as he stopped all to talk.
Astonished gasps filled the air, as the peasant man
saw only their same level, he now could not understand.

"Won't you let us in, and won't you let us stay?
We've suffered a forest fire, which has blown our house away.
We won't cause you any trouble, that I promise you,
as you never in our house, which once stood well and true".

What other statement could turn such upper heads,
as the Jeevis household, embarrassed, but furiously said:
"Master Grace, please escort these dear people to the door".

Along with the look of 'please don't come and
visit here any more!'

How could such a man turn such an incident
away?
How could Grace, who became a pal also,
know just what he could say?
They saved his life, gave them a home and
freedom for a while,
but due only to the upper friend's thoughts,
had he to turn so vile.

So they roamed hungry and cold, and with
nowhere to lie.
When one day announced that family pauper
had to die.
They could not go back, so they stayed in
that town's rich face,
where the Jeevis mansion could, but did not
offer a place.

When the bulletin of the family hit the news,
there was only one guilty family to accuse.
Witnesses from the party came forward to
declare,
that the family once knew the Jeevis name,
for they were there.

Every Jeevis member went to visit the scruffy
morgue,
in that old shanty town where they had visited
before.

Looks were upon their dead faces as if to say
but not to moan,
"We'd invite you back for coffee, but we
haven't got a home!"

20 Sometimes It Takes

Sometimes it takes
such a whopping great mistake,
for someone to see,
or to become the good hearted.
It may have to be
in the form of a tragedy,
in order for them to now appreciate
what they before took for granted.

Sometimes it takes
a gust of wind or an earthquake,
to see things differently,
or to become a better person,
to open closed eyes,
or wake up to realise.
A situation needs to take its place
to teach a lesson in a different version.

At first you may get
a gentle whisper in the head,
then a small gale,
then a hurricane full-blown.
How long will we wait,
until we choose which one to take?
While matters increase and worsen,
how many danger signals must be shown?

Where will we choose
to step off, before the blown fuse?
In life's such hazards,

if we can help them, then let's halt them.
The longer the loose brick lies around,
the sooner the whole house will fall down.
I'd rather catch the subtle breeze's warning,
but maybe for some, that's not enough that's
taught them.

Alec Alcoholic
didn't stop at gin and tonic.
His warning light had flashed blindingly
in his early stages.
It had to take one drink more
before it hit home with the score.
And sooner than he knew it,
he was pushing up the daisies.

Susie Sleeparound
frequently stepped on danger ground.
Her attention wasn't caught.
To the AIDS scare, she didn't listen.
One HIV,
another two, another three.
How many more increased chances should it
take
for her to be frightened out of her position?

21 It Takes One To Know One
(Blessing in Disguise)

for Ash

Twenty years ago this week
saw the tragic scene.
How she thought she'd never speak
of it's happening.
Today she runs the busy centre
of the rape crisis.
An offering to all who enter,
who've experienced like this.

It was ten years ago today,
he was the tragic case.
How he thought he'd never say
how alcohol defaced.
Today he lectures everywhere
of the drink crisis.
An offering to all who care,
who experience like this.

It takes one to know one,
and sometimes misfortune
can be of help to grow one
out of their mess too.
At the time, their tragedy.
At present, their motive.
Taken then to agony
for a destiny to give.

22 Souls Out To Serve

We would be led into believing ideas
that contradict truths
and our wide open ears.
It stands to our reason
as an answer to prayer,
but the answer to us
may in disagreeable form be there.

God, we acknowledge as the head of all
control.
His people are painful,
yet numb are his souls.
Used are the spirits
when finished with their nerves.
His people on trial.
His souls out to serve.

Guardian angels surround us in need.
The highest determines
which one plucks the weed.
Working through his fine creation
of the souls.
Claiming them back
from their bodies pierced with holes.

When the flesh lived, it suffered it's torment
in it's specified trauma
that earth's life had sent.
So when the shell leaves
the hurting and the pain,
that soul can drum it's energy

into helping the same.

Placing itself in a task to do well,
the deceased alcoholic
can assist the living drunk now.
Our guardian angels
of their past experience,
have since rid their trouble,
when freed from bodily existence.

Selected for us, for individual circumstance,
there's one for each wound
to heal for our preference.
So when we pass by our bruise,
likewise for another with the same,
we'll be at their side supporting,
although they won't know we came.

So now in our lifetime of harassment and
scars,
let us begin to acknowledge
where the unseen folk are.
Their motives for us
as our spiritual guides
will duly be our purpose
when we've reached the other side.

23 (This Is) Where I Lived Before I Was Born

It's not the dream you have
where when you wake – it's all gone.
It's not the dream
where every detail's in its place, but one's
wrong.
I remember waking in the night
from the loud cry that awoke me.
I remember putting up the fight
with that voice which gagged and choked me.

It's kind of embarrassing
explaining to a chosen few.
How do you tell good friends convincingly
that merely a dream is true?
Since my mind was forced to learn of a one
time residence,
I checked it out of curiosity,
to reveal my past lifetime's experience
dwelled here to disprove my set philosophy.

Every detail
from the layout to the era was correct.
All its surrounding probed my memory
to find what it should expect.
Recollections of centuries ago,
not impractical mental imagery.
In this house I watched my children grow.
On this lawn I held the local village tea.

Sometimes I look back

at the life I had before this one replaced.
A different gender was I then,
as was the difference in my race.
Sharing with them is now something that I
leave.
They mock and dodge and scorn.
I'll just satisfy myself with the truth that I
believe,
in knowing this is where I lived before I was
born.

24 Counting On The Guidance

Ruby glances at me with Satan in her eyes.
She will mock me.
She will ridicule my belief I've been raised on
for nearly all of my life,
though I tell her of my Jesus story.
I want this sinful child of God to repent of her
evil way.
She will not listen, but only rebuke all I say.

Parted are we from our condemned
relationship.
So unnatural,
so unintended says my Saviour who convicts
me,
he who tells me that he will have to punish it.
I'm left angry, so I drift away
from this huge Creator who made me the
way that I am.
How can they turn 'round to tell me that he
understands?

Ruby calls me with LSD in her eyes,
knives in her wrists,
and repentance in her mind.
Counting on my guidance,
but the blind are leading the blind,
even though she seeks this God given
Samaritan
with previous gifts of spiritual need.
Never before had she requested to accept
this Christ to bleed.

Knock knock. Who's there? Well, I'm not
here anymore.
Known no longer at this ancient address.
I have moved out while she's searching,
but nothing's there at my door.
I feel useless, I feel angry
knowing fault isn't with God,
but rather the blame's down to me.
For her sanity's sake why have I become
God's divorcee?

She's asking questions I can't provide
answers for.
I no longer can give personal opinion.
I know what I'm supposed to say,
but don't believe it any more.
Words from lips contradict a heart that's
beating
unrighteousness where information such as
this fails.
Something or someone off track must be
replaced on the rails.

Ruby tells me, had she known that God I'd
left,
never would she have made contact,
only to find the support she needed
lived no more in my nest.
Years back she would have gained sermons
from me,
but since then my testing time has gripped
the better of me.

It's been a long stretch since I lived with him,
as he with me.

I'm the last one to go religious on you,
but I can't believe God allowed you
to survive after your near death
to repeat what you've been put through.
Still you claim this as your punishment due.
I can't turn my back on someone who's
turned towards me.
Hard as I fight this, I love you unconditionally.

While you're dealing and coming to terms
with all of this,
how I'm learning,
how myself I have to cope with your new leaf
you've turned
and the suicide you've missed.
You delved too deeply into my hollow heart,
but I guess desperation time prefers
comforting words,
than hard opinions believed in which should
remain unheard.

Ruby, how I wish you every success
with your fresh life,
with your Lord who saved you.
How I wish I also could be there with you
blessed,
and how I wished I could have rearranged
you.
Don't you agree it's a strange fact to be now
we've moved along?

Our roles have changed, your soul's
gained, while mine's deprived and wrong.

25 Waiting For The Anti-Christ

I've been such a good boy
from December to December,
but I've been so conned into believing in this
false prophet
from ever since I can remember.
But I'm still laying here quietly and
expectantly.
I'm waiting for the Anti-Christ
to come a-shootin' down the chimney
in his smart suit of Satan red,
while I'm faking sleep and faith,
tucked up in my 'good boy' bed.
I'm waiting for the Anti-Christ
to come a-shootin' down the chimney.
I'll tell him who's the Boss,
as I rebel from the presence he's sent.

He's the conman who will trick us in the
middle of the night.
Who leaves us feeling proud
by our well earned goodness,
and then disappears out of sight.
But we're all still laying here so naive, while
he deceives,
waiting for the Anti-Christ
to come a-shootin' down the chimney
in his smart suit of Satan red.
I read
that many would come

claiming the name of the person he's stood in
for.
So now I'm telling you, Santa Claus,
that there's no room at my chimney's inn
door.
So now we're forced to see baby Jesus
wrapped under a totally different disguise.
He's somehow all grown old now,
awaiting for Christmas Eve's gift from every
child,
of a carrot for his transport,
and for himself, a hot mince pie.
Yes, he's stepped right in to stand in his
place.
Do we see this holy day's whole reasoning
as a white haired old man's face?
It's the pure newborn baby's celebration day
only,
so Santa's sell by date must be passed,
for Jesus Christ can't be reduced for quick
sale,
due to the purpose of his task.

So I'm waiting for the Anti-Christ
to come a-shootin' down the chimney
in his smart suit of Satan red,
to give him the chance to let me pass on
what a good boy I've been.
I'll let him know that I don't have to earn any
more
to show how I've been accepted into the
truth,
by requesting and being redeemed.

The yearly pass won't eternally last,
but the life long one will,
from the truth of the Christmas scene.

26   Shameless Friend

Hello there shameless friend,
on fire for the Lord.
Your faith and your twin blade sword
may just well offend.
The 'born—again' remarks.
Christ Jesus crucified.
How soon are they to bark.
How is their God of lies?!
Gonna get this Holy girl.
Gonna break me out of sin.
Gonna get this Holy girl-
Holy girl to break me in.

Hello there Trinity-
your tongue is getting stale,
as I hammer another nail
into the hands that set me free.
Well, Jesus you never robbed
a woman's sacred touch.
Your embrace can't make me throb.
Your distaste don't account for much.
Gonna get this Holy girl.
Gonna break me out of sin.
Gonna get this Holy girl-
Holy girl come break me in.

27 A Mass Flight Into Space
(Last Piece Of The Puzzle)

God light surrounding to glow
the chosen few that you should know.
Cupped by hands, together bound.
The unbelievers' vision scoffs.
Doubter hanging on the edge
of the hand destined to pledge.
Climbs onto the finger small,
only to be shaken off.

Earth not as yet seen the last
let alone the first, peeked by the vast.
The final view of Jesus Christ
will not be one in weakness.
A reversal in this picture concerned.
Piercings of strength hold his return,
not as Saviour this time around,
rather as the Ruler crowned.

The world's biggest sensation
beamed on every TV station.
'The Missing Millions' reads headline.
One to firmly pitch us.
How the world will then respond;
"We don't quite know what happened,
but their common factor stands;
they were all 'religious'!"

Sceptic scoffers forever humming;
"Where's the promise of his coming?"
God's gracious plan of love vows

to be perfect and honest.
Lengthening out the day of grace,
unwilling that any should perish and waste,
but all would come to repentance.
Not slack in concerning his promise.

Prophecy is the Bible's proof
that the Bible is the truth.
Certainty is guaranteed
in the Holy Scripture.
What the 'high' books have to say,
how the influences stray,
education disobeys,
to distort the clearest picture.

His Majesty's second advent
is mentioned more than when first sent.
The day lies hid, that every day
we be watchful and wise.
Living each day like it were
when his return will occur.
Keeping us Holy and to
urgently evangelise.

Like a thief he'll arrive, (our sin slave),
robbing the world of its saved,
like a big surprise unannounced,
while the world is sleeping.
Totally casual, totally unprepared,
a world troubled by tragic affairs,
but the last thing on it's mind
will be this visitor's greeting.

What a mess he'll come back to clear out.
No wonder he's coming with a shout.
Many will jump from not hearing about
this momentous occasion.
Drugging themselves into oblivion,
losing what they could have won,
leaving salvation undone
to face this dreadful invasion.

Light and salt gone, Hell let loose.
Mark of the Beast introduced.
We now have technology
to track every person.
Those who took this Christ to receive,
further than history's fact believed,
have escaped found,
but the lost have escaped God's version.

In the twinkling of an eye,
into space this mass will fly
with him, and I will deny
this as an unlikely story.
Alone, this ship world would not float,
but thank God Christ's the lifeboat.
Thank God, death is swallowed up
in this great victory.

The plot currently incomplete,
awaiting the rest to take its seat.
The second arrival paints
the whole picture clearly.
The Earth must cease its beating heart,
to begin eternity's start.

If Satan reminds you of your past,
remind him that his future's dreary!

28 Planet Zoor

A little man from planet Zoor came rushing to
his friends,
to tell that he had been to Earth,
and to let them know our trends.
Well, the Zoorites said;
"He's cracked up now, he's just escaped from
his mind!"
So little Zoorlot wandered home,
and hoped one day that they'd find.
"They've got these beings called 'people'
there,
they have two arms and legs".
But they just didn't believe or care.
"They've only got one head", he said.
"They also have these objects which fly.
I think they're called aeroplanes.
They go real high up in the sky.
They've also got computer games".
The Zoorites laughed and laughed once
more,
as poor old Zoorlot claimed;
that if he was in their shoes right then,
he would have done the same.
"How I wish I could take you there,
but I don't know the way.
I wish you could see these humans,
it's so funny how they play".

Well, they don't believe,
because their minds can't accept.

They're brought up in that way.
They don't know any differently.
They're not us.
And that's the way it may always stay.
"It's a fairy tale", they say.
There must be a much bigger being
to create them in that way.
What they don't realise is that humans made
them up from far away.
"We're one step higher from them", we say.

Do you believe me when I say that a man will
come from the sky,
and only take the ones who love him
to live with him way up high?
Well, you may say that I've cracked up now,
and I've just escaped from my mind!
So now I'll just wander back home,
and hope one day that you'll find.
They've got these beings called 'angels'
there.
They're clad in white and have wings.
But you just don't believe or care.
They've even got a voice which sings.
They worship too the one in the sky.
The one who I said will come.
Why waste your time on wondering why,
when you can get to know the Son?
The humans laughed and laughed once
more,
as poor old I still claim;
that if I was in their shoes right then,
I would have made a change.

How I wish I could take you there,
but for you I don't know the way.
I wish you could see what I see,
because it's so sad the way you play.

Well, they don't believe,
because their minds can't accept.
They're brought up in that way.
They don't know any differently.
We're not God,
and that's the way it will always stay.
So, "it's a fairy tale", they say.
There surely must be a much bigger being to
make us in this way.
What some don't realise is that our Creator
made us up from far away.
"He's one step higher from us", I say.

29 Supernatural Crowds

Year after year you inform me
of how Mary's visitor appeared.
You believe of what you've been told,
but not of what you hear.
The everlasting energy of my killed son
revealed itself, much to your disbelief.
But I'm no chosen one,
and it was the outcome of my grief!

'Jesus will return soon',
you state so adamantly.
Yet you snigger at her perfect claim;
'That Angel was seen so visibly'.
When the trumpet blasts,
and he's way above us,
will you still say that it's just the clouds!?
Maybe he's shown how to love us,
through supernatural crowds.

We're expected to believe in what we've simply
been told.
Yet we have to ignore the signs.
A distortion of the truth will misguide your soul.
The enemy is set to blind.
The paranormal can't hold joy.
If not safely held within the scripture alone,
we must avoid and destroy.
As Mary, we must stone.

You flaunt your faith in God that you feel,
so don't kill the God that I've seen.

God doesn't die at Revelation.
And upon faith relies the unseen.
No tampering with spirit guides and the
deceased.
The clinically dead have lived to tell.
Their loved ones upon Earth who had
disbelieved,
seem to be there as well.

30 Science is only the stuff that man can reach!

There has to have been a point in time
where life was breathed into the whole of
existence.
Out of nothing comes nothing.
Something enabled life's assistance.
Chemicals clashing,
explosions flashing. They do not have a
mind!
A big bang alone can't be responsible for it,
can it?!
It's common sense to believe
that we didn't put ourselves on this planet!

We don't want to use this swear word, 'God',
Are we afraid of having to limit him to one
fixed abode?
An energy outside of human existence must
exist,
or we would remain in darkness mode,
as was the same
before the explosion of light came.
Does it not make perfect sense?!
It all falls hand in hand in its clear indication.
What more can God do to prove himself,
when we've closed our minds from
persuasion?!

If we arrived by chance only,
wouldn't other things happen by chance too?!
Are we mistakes then?

We get freak conditions, but they are few.
Not enough to understand
that we're unplanned.
Other things don't take place by chance.
What knows that the skeleton must grow the
same rate as the flesh?
Our development is mapped.
What knows we have to eat? Food's here by
chance I guess!!

Scientifically, energy can never die.
We are water and dust but also emotion and
memory,
for what the physically seen matter alone
takes no responsibility.
Chemicals clashing,
explosions flashing.
A mind comes behind creation.
There's a whole lot more to life than what we
can humanly see.
There's a whole lot more to life
and to complex you and me!

The reason man will never discover God,
is not because he's not there, but because
he's beyond science.
Just because science can't prove,
we mustn't dismiss life's unfathomed giants!
Can't put love or hate
into a test tube and wait
for it's existence in a lab.
Yet we believe in emotion, just as God, we
can't physically detect.

God is before and after science.
Man has much to find within the universe as
yet!

We have animals that sense what we cannot
detect.
Because we can't see invisible company
clear
surrounding us by our human eye,
doesn't mean to say that they're not here!
You say I've been brainwashed into believing
what I believe in, in receiving. But it works
both ways;
Have I been brainwashed with Christianity as
much as you have with psychology?!
Every time you point the finger at me,
three point back at you with no apology!

It's interesting that you don't often hear of
athiests
that have experienced the paranormal or
supernatural.
Who have witnessed faith or ghosts.
You cannot disprove another's case that's
factual.
There's too much evidence
of supernatural events.
The whole concept of God
and life after death is way beyond wishful
flatteries,
but in the majority, an inbuilt common sense.
we leave our shells behind
rather than fizzle out like batteries!

There's too much spiritual backup
for it all to be simple bare.
You're making two and two make seven.
You're not looking at what's blatantly there!
You're looking way ahead.
You're lost where you've been lead.
Man has to be the highest.
He demands all the answers, he can't make
room for question marks.
They simply won't do.
But now tell me, what breathed life at the
start?!

Things don't enable or create themselves.
We can still have evolved by what the
almighty has grown.
The day that man makes a man,
Not reproduces or clones,
but takes the raw ingredients,
and breathes in him obedience,
and forms him as his own,
as Frankenstein's creator, that's the day I
panic and surrender,
and become an atheist-
living life as the average contender!

31 God's shaking his head

I tuck her in.
She prays, 'sorry for her sin'.
She says, 'I hate this Jesus,
he never lets you do anything!
'No no darling, don't say any more.
Jesus says, 'let's change the law,
so that we can live'.
It's the nasty people who claim to love him
who don't love him at all!'

The Gospel according to 'us'
is a safe scripture to trust.
If we don't like insanity
we call it a sin, we call it a lust.
Even the 'forward' to the book of light
says, 'we've tried our hardest to get it right
just remember, we are little man!'
I want to see the grey show up
between the black and white.
I want to see the difference
between what's really wrong and right!

I'm far away
from all that's near, I'm all astray.
I've never heard of the man
with the golden ticket to lead the way.
On God territory
I feel many things in me.
I make many mistakes.
I can't believe because it says believe-
I have intellect you see.

We're told we're not perfect,
but what can't be proved, if we don't accept
we pay 'big time' for apparently,
if we don't know that we're in dept.
I find it rather odd
to worship an 'ogre' 'schizoidal' God,
who will cast into Hell fire
through unrecognition of the one-way
system,
or not knowing when to nod.

One book stationed;
not only different denominations
of the top prize faith,
but we've runners up: all the different
relations.
Billy Grahams vision soars,
Billy Idols same one flaws!
I don't understand,
when we all entered God's world as equals,
of some we take note more.

I'd rather face
my worn out brain all over the place,
than have a simple faith
trusting God will find my parking space!
I'll go walking around town,
clad in sandwich board and dressing gown,
with my odd shoes on.
Reeking with digestive biscuits, claiming to
be the messiah,
'AND I'M COMING BACK RIGHT NOW!!!'

God's shaking his head,
in his hands once whipped and bled.
Saying; 'this isn't what I planned,
I wanna go home, go to bed!
and I hope you sort it out, take it up
amongst yourselves and wake up!!!
I'm not gonna move,
but you keep shunting me around,
by the 'God-given' nature of your human
make-up.

32 Truths From Untruths

Well, we've been waiting far too long now.
I believe it's now time to confess.
So I'm gonna take you on a trip to view
the mystery behind Monroe's death.
Then we'll travel a little further,
to wipe out the whole of Loch Ness.
We're gonna pick up all our questions.
We're gonna put them to the test.

We're gonna freeze out in the cold,
and that Yeti, we will find.
Then we'll return to the Hendrix Hotel,
to see if it was really suicide.
And regarding this human combustion,
it's truth will now be clarified.
And if we produce no evidence,
at least we will have tried.

We'll persevere in hunting for that
unfathomed UFO,
and when returned to Earth, spot Elvis
shopping in Tesco.
We'll suss out all these mysteries,
so we can then know
the truths from the untruths.
We'll put their evidence on show.

33 Proportion Of Existence

Trying to conceive the child.
You've no idea how long it takes.
My body's clock is ticking away,
so I can't afford the wait.
No matter where I turn,
what stays refusing to leave
is pregnancy surrounding me
like you would not believe.
You know, I just can't shake those
antenatal classes advertised
off my sleeve.

Trying to come to terms,
but her death rules in my head.
My memories are in present tense.
No, I can't accept her dead.
No matter where I turn,
what stays refusing to leave
is death surrounding me
like you would not believe.
You know, I just can't shake those
hearses, wreaths and graves of everyday
off my sleeve.

Trying to meet the man,
but a husband I can't find.
My pure white dress is fading with time,
unlike the idea in my mind.
No matter where I turn,
what stays refusing to leave
is marriage surrounding me

like you would not believe.
You know, I just can't shake those
brides and grooms smiles upon their faces
off my sleeve.

Trying to get so hard
what life just doesn't bring
seems to be increased
within our surrounding.
No matter where we turn,
we see it more through sensitivity.
Our awareness of it becomes broader
than one's who isn't bothered by its intensity.
Its proportion of existence
has always been the very same,
despite the compulsion to expand,
held within our capability.

34 A Place Where Life Is Ideal.
A Place Freed From The Cell

There's a girl called Fran,
the proud owner of the Down's syndrome.
Her mind's almost everywhere
except in home.
She's never lived reality.
In fantasy she's dressed,
all locked in her head,
but tell me, which way's best?

There's a woman named Maude,
convinced she's in line to the throne.
Dementia trusts her Royalty.
In this, she's on her own.
How absolutely awesome to die
believing you are who you claim to be.
Is this pathetic and sad?
How great to cease in insanity!

There's a man, he's fully grown,
yet he's re-acting his infancy.
Babyism's answer avoids responsibility.
Adulthood escapism
appears to be only through death's door.
So is this perverted and sick?
Do we never feel this insecure?

Expand your dream,
however far, however wide.
Don't allow reality's limits
to make you hide.

Only fairytale joy enters
wherever it chooses to dwell.
A place where life is ideal.
A place freed from the cell.

If these three gemstones
live life that's just as real,
why is it a shame life's lacked ,
or is it, still?
Maybe you're the one who's lost out on
the boundaries life can break through.
It's all very well to pity them,
while they've more reason to pity you!

35 The Process Of Our Foreign Kingdom

Crazy cats sniff the butts of their members.
Dozy dogs lick the faces of men.
We respect the process of our foreign
kingdom,
but dare the Boss to make that move again!
The human race is so reserved to say the
least.
Our physical affection surrenders all unto the
beast.
Sometimes I can't help but envy our fellow
creature's action.
Sometimes I can't help but believe we've got
it wrong.

How nice it would be to have your head feel
stroked,
when at the bus stop you're casually sat.
Or in the tense waiting room of the dentist,
you could curl up on somebody's lap.
Imagine queuing hours on end just to get
served.
How short the time would seem if only we
were not so reserved.
I'm sure our beasty chums view ours as such
a tragic case.
Breakdowns and traumas yearn affection to
replace.

36 I Am, So Don't (Just Recognise)

I am an individual – a single.
I am a non-mover – a non-mingle.
I am one parented – a fatherless off-springle.
So don't marry me,
don't carry me,
don't daddy me.

I am a slowcoach – a time taker.
I am a concern – a panic maker.
I am a living flesh – a dead meat faker.
So don't hurry me,
don't worry me,
don't curry me.

You are a pest – an intrusion.
I am a non-affectionate – a hugger's illusion.
I am a mess – a confusion.
So don't trouble me,
don't cuddle me,
don't muddle me.

I am a non-existent – an abortion.
I am a wariness symbol – a caution.
I am a liar – a truth distortion.
So don't conceive me,
don't receive me,
don't believe me.

I am a lunatic – a mad man,
I am a rotter – a bad man,
I am a weeper – a sad man.

So don't pester me,
don't mess with me,
don't depress me.

If you are quiet – don't shout it.
If you are positive – don't doubt it.
If you are needy – don't go without it.
Don't try to change,
don't rearrange,
don't confuse names.
Don't disorganise,
don't criticise,
just recognise.

37 Aspects For Prejudice

Like the thug,
he relies on fists.
Like the bigot,
he relies on prejudice.
Like the black versus the white skin.
Like the Hindu versus the Christian origin.
Like the heterosexual who versus the
homosexual preference.
And when we've finished battling,
we're still left with their difference.

Like the puzzle
that is never solved.
Like the bitter pill
that is never dissolved.
Like the religion that is anti-gay.
Like the race against the celebrated day.
Like both disagreeing sides
of each topic mentioned previously,
we're now battling with subject difference,
by category versus category.

It's one minority
attacking another minority
and it really stinks.
It's one prejudice
attacking another prejudice
where only bigotry thinks.
It's the forcing of issues and opinions,
in the aim to intrude a personal belief,

and you know when that equivalent is
sexually concerned,
it's then being raped by the beast.

With the enemy,
a friend can't be there.
With a forced friendship,
there's never a two sided affair.
With harassment,
a person is pushed against will.
With the conflict,
no side of the wound can be healed
With both side's consequence never reaching
the same conclusion,
we have to agree to differ,
and not become our brother's intrusion.

Unlike the foe,
let us tolerate our opposition.
Unlike the inconsiderate,
let us raise the proposition
to dislike stubbornness and the concept of
enemy.
Unlike having to like.
we don't have to hate,
in order to disagree,
unlike our world how it shamefully stands
with it's outcasts and it's rejections.
Let us introduce equality unconditionally,
with it's prospect for all - acceptance.
You see, we don't have to agree
in order to keep the peace.

We just accept that our opposition is merely
our opponent's opinion,
enabling the warfare to cease.

38 Social Misfit

Every school community
consists of the 'faggot' he's been termed.
Their attention for opportunity
has been divided to not learn
those subjects their concentration
should be directed at,
but they'd rather waste their intellect,
creating victims from the esteem they lack.

Every close knit neighbourhood
consists of the 'odd-ball' character.
Their tongues and fingers wagging
teams up their actors and amateurs.
Those issues their consideration
should be directed at,
has been exchanged for boredom,
creating victims from the esteem they lack.

Every office environment
consists of the religious freak's insanity.
Their equally entitled opinion
can't take this Christianity.
Those morals their condemnation
should be directed at,
have the substitute of bigotry,
creating victims from the knowledge they
lack.

Every small minority
that doesn't fit the scene,
stands on the outside looking in

at a majority cold and mean.
Every small minority
disagreeing with their next,
has their neighbour down for opponent,
creating victims from that group they've
assessed.

Acceptance is a virtue
owed to all humanity.
Each person must learn
to respect individuality,
and every person in their right
is uniquely designed.
Is your neighbour your opponent?
Are you creating victims?
Have you the narrow mind?

www.ingramcontent.com/pod-product-compliance
Lightning Source LLC
Chambersburg PA
CBHW031217270326
41931CB00006B/591